Post Kidney Transplant Recovery and Diet Guide

With **20** Recipes for Smooth Healing.

By
CYNTHIA LEONARD

TABLE OF CONTENTS

TABLE OF CONTENTS   2

INTRODUCTION   6

    OVERVIEW OF THE RECOVERY PROCESS   9

    PREPARING FOR THE JOURNEY   13

CHAPTER 1: Pre-Transplant Nutrition Guidelines   17

    PSYCHOLOGICAL PREPARATION FOR THE TRANSPLANT 20

    POST-TRANSPLANT NUTRITION BASICS   22

CHAPTER 2: Dietary Restrictions and Recommendations   25

    Post - Kidney Transplant   25

    FLUID INTAKE GUIDELINES   28

    BUILDING A HEALTHY PLATE   30

CHAPTER 3: Portion Control and Meal Frequency   33

    CONTROLLED PORTION   33

FREQUENCY OF MEALS   35

MEAL PLANNING FOR RECOVERY   37

    Things to Think About: 39

    Safety Measures: 39

CHAPTER 4: Understanding the Interaction Between
Immunosuppressants and Diet   41

    TIMING MEALS AND MEDICATIONS   44

    ADDRESSING COMMON CHALLENGES   45

CHAPTER 5: Dealing with Taste Changes and Appetite
Fluctuations   51

    COPING WITH DIGESTIVE ISSUES   52

CHAPTER 6: Physical Activity and Wellness   54

    INCORPORATING EXERCISE INTO THE RECOVERY
    ROUTINE   54

    STRESS MANAGEMENT STRATEGIES   55

CHAPTER 7: Adapting Nutritional Habits for
Sustainable Health   60

Periodic Nutritional Assessments and Adjustments   61

20 Nutrient-Rich Recipes   65

**20 POST KIDNEY TRANSPLANT RECIPES THAT HELPS
DURING YOUR HEALING PROCESS.**   66

BREAKFAST   66

LUNCH   78

DINNER   90

SNACKS   102

**MEAL PLANNER FOR DIFFERENT DIETARY NEEDS.
112**

INTRODUCTION

People's general health and well-being are greatly influenced by their diet and this is - especially the case for people who have had kidney transplants.

Following a kidney transplant, eating a healthy diet is crucial to promoting the healing process, preserving organ function and avoiding problems.

The following are some major points underscoring the significance of diet after a kidney transplant:

Immune System Support: To avoid their new kidney being rejected, transplant patients often take immunosuppressive drugs. These drugs have the potential to impair immunity, increasing a person's susceptibility to illnesses. An immune system boosting, infection-prevention diet high in vitamins, minerals and antioxidants may help maintain a well-balanced diet.

Wound Healing and Recovery: Even in cases when surgery goes well, the body may experience stress. Sufficient nourishment is essential for healthy wound healing and recuperation. Particularly, protein is necessary for tissue regeneration and eating a diet high in protein helps hasten the healing process.

Bone Health: Certain post-transplant drugs, such corticosteroids, may be detrimental to bone health. Vitamin D and calcium are two nutrients that are crucial for keeping strong, healthy bones. Dairy products, leafy greens and meals fortified with nutrients are good sources of calcium for the diet.

Blood Pressure Control: Heart-healthy, low-sodium diets may help control blood pressure, which is prevalent in kidney transplant patients. Reducing consumption of canned products, processed meals and high-sodium snacks is part of this.

Diabetes management: People who get transplants may be more likely to acquire diabetes. For those with diabetes, a balanced diet that controls blood sugar levels is essential. It might be helpful to keep an eye on your carbohydrate consumption and to choose complex carbs over simple sweets.

Fluid Balance: Kidney function depends on enough fluid intake. Recipients of transplants may need to keep an eye on their fluid intake to avoid dehydration or overload, depending on their specific situation and medicines.

Reducing Drug Side Effects: A few drugs have the potential to have adverse effects including weight gain or lipid level alterations. Regular exercise and a balanced diet may improve cardiovascular health and aid in weight management.

Preventing Metabolic Syndrome: High blood pressure, high cholesterol and abdominal obesity are among the components of metabolic syndrome that may be brought on by long-term use of immunosuppressive drugs. These risk factors can be managed with a balanced diet.

Kidney transplant patients should collaborate closely with healthcare providers, such as nutritionists or dietitians to customise their diets according to their unique medical conditions, prescription drugs and nutritional demands.

Long-term kidney transplant success may be greatly increased by maintaining a healthy lifestyle, according to medical advice and receiving regular monitoring.

OVERVIEW OF THE RECOVERY PROCESS

An important stage that comes after the surgical operation of kidney transplantation is the kidney transplant recovery process. How well the recipient's body absorbs the new kidney and how well they handle the postoperative care will determine whether or not the transplant is successful.

This is a summary of the recuperation period after a kidney transplant:

1. The immediate postoperative period *(hospital stay)*:

Length: Depending on the patient's health, the first hospital stay usually lasts between five and ten days.

Monitoring: In the first few hours after surgery, a close eye is kept on the patient's vital signs and kidney function.

Immune Suppression: To stop the immune system from attacking the new kidney, recipients are given immunosuppressive drugs.

2. Monitoring and Follow-Up:

Outpatient Visits: Following discharge, patients must see the transplant team on a regular basis to have their kidney function, medication levels and general health checked.

Lab testing: To evaluate kidney function and the efficacy of immunosuppressive medications, blood tests, such as those measuring creatinine levels, are routinely carried out.

3. Medication Management:

Immunosuppressive Drugs: Immunosuppressive drug usage must be continued for the rest of one's life in order to avoid organ rejection. Medication kinds and dosages may change over time.

Anti-Rejection Drugs: Anti-rejection medications such as corticosteroids, mycophenolate mofetil and tacrolimus are often administered.

4. Lifestyle and Diet: In order to maintain kidney function and effectively manage medicine, recipients may need to adhere to a certain diet.

Hydration: Sustaining enough fluids is critical for kidney health.

Exercise: As recommended by healthcare professionals, gradually increase your physical activity level.

5. Prophylactic Medication for Infection Prevention: Antibiotics or antiviral drugs may be recommended to stop infections.

Immunisations: Depending on the patient's immunosuppressed status, a few vaccines may be advised to strengthen the immune system.

6. Emotional and Mental Health:

Support Groups: Attending support groups for transplant recipients may provide insightful information as well as emotional assistance.

Psychological Support: Following a transplant, some people may have emotional difficulties. Counselling and psychosocial assistance might be helpful.

7. Getting Back to Your Regular Activities:

Job and Life: The timeline for going back to work and engaging in daily activities varies depending on the patient's overall level of recuperation.

Physical rehabilitation involves gradually increasing exercise to build back strength.

8. Extended-Term Care: Continuous Monitoring For the remainder of the recipient's life, routine examinations and kidney function monitoring are carried out.

Medication Adherence: In order to avoid rejection, strict adherence to prescribed medication regimens is necessary.

Difficulties and Turndowns: Keeping an eye out for complications Frequent examinations assist in detecting and treating any possible issues.

Signals of Rejection: Patients are informed about the warning signals of rejection, which include elevated creatinine levels and flu-like symptoms and are advised to see a doctor right once if they manifest.

It's vital to remember that everyone's recuperation process is unique and for the best results, constant coordination with the transplant team is essential.

PREPARING FOR THE JOURNEY

A number of crucial procedures must be followed in order to guarantee a successful and seamless kidney transplant procedure. This is a broad overview; however, individual experiences may differ, so it's important to speak with your healthcare team for specific recommendations:

Consultation and Assessment:

Collaborate carefully with your medical team to determine if a kidney transplant is required.
Go through a comprehensive assessment to find out whether you qualify for a transplant. This covers exams related to health, psychology and finances.

Finding a Donor:

Find family members and acquaintances who could be willing live donors. As an alternative, you could be added to a kidney donor waiting list. Examine the eligibility of the donor and do compatibility testing.

Budgetary Management:

Recognise the expenses of kidney transplantation, including the cost of the procedure, the drugs, the aftercare and any problems. Examine your choices for financial aid and insurance.

Counselling and Education:

Attend instructional classes to get knowledge about possible hazards, post-transplant care and the transplant procedure, because receiving a kidney transplant may be a difficult process, seek out counselling for psychological and emotional support.

Screening and Immunisation before to transplantation:

To determine your general health, have all necessary medical exams and screenings completed.

To reduce the chance of infections after the transplant, make sure all vaccines are current.

Sustaining Maximum Well-Being:

Prior to the transplant, maintain a healthy lifestyle that includes a balanced diet and frequent exercise. Control long-term health issues, including diabetes or high blood pressure, to minimise consequences.

Management of Medication:

Talk to your healthcare provider about the medicines you're taking now, since some may need to be changed or stopped.

Recognise the post-transplant drug schedule, which usually consists of immunosuppressants to avoid rejection.

Planning Logistics:

Make travel plans to and from the transplant facility. Make travel and lodging arrangements in advance, as you might need to spend the healing phase close to the hospital.

Solid Support System:

Create a solid support network of friends and family who can offer both practical and emotional support during the transplant process.

After-transplant Care:

Recognise the significance of post-transplant care, which includes following prescribed dosage schedules, getting regular checkups and keeping an eye out for rejection symptoms.

Recall that having an optimistic outlook, following your healthcare team's advice and maintaining open lines of communication can all help ensure a successful kidney transplant experience.

CHAPTER 1: Pre-Transplant Nutrition Guidelines

Maintaining a healthy diet prior to a kidney transplant is essential for supporting general health and getting the body ready for the procedure. But it's important to remember that every person has different dietary requirements, so detailed recommendations should be tailored to the patient's health, stage of renal disease and other circumstances.

For individualised guidance, always speak with a medical professional or a qualified dietitian.

The following basic dietary recommendations apply before a kidney transplant:

Regulate Blood Sugar and Blood Pressure:

Keep your blood pressure and blood sugar under rigorous control since uncontrolled diabetes and hypertension may have a detrimental effect on kidney function.

Consumption of Protein:

Depending on the stage of renal illness, modify your protein consumption. Depending on the individual's health state, a modest protein restriction may be advised in certain situations.

Fluid Consumption:

To prevent dehydration or excessive fluid retention, keep an eye on and regulate your fluid intake. Guidelines tailored to your individual requirements will be provided by your healthcare team.

Electrolytes:

Make sure that your levels of potassium, phosphorus, and sodium are adequate. Based on your test findings, a nutritionist will advise you on what foods to include or avoid.

Vitamin D and Calcium:

Make sure you're getting enough calcium and vitamin D to maintain healthy bones. Given that renal illness may impact bone metabolism, this is very crucial.

Controlling Weight:

Reach and maintain a healthy weight. Although controlling one's weight is important, drastic or crash diets should be avoided.

Limit Consumption of Sodium:

Limit your salt consumption to support fluid balance and blood pressure management. This entails cutting down on meals rich in sodium and staying away from additional salt.

Tailored Dietary Programme:

Create a customised nutrition plan with the help of a certified dietitian that takes into account your lifestyle, food choices, and unique medical condition.

Management of Medication:

As directed by your healthcare team, take your medicines as directed and talk to your doctor about any possible dietary interactions or side effects.

Food safety and Cleanliness:

To lower the risk of infections, practise excellent hygiene and food safety. This might be especially crucial for those with weakened immune systems.

Do note that these are just broad suggestions; tailored dietary advice is mandatory. A licensed dietician as part of your healthcare team will evaluate your individual requirements and provide recommendations in line with those findings.

PSYCHOLOGICAL PREPARATION FOR THE TRANSPLANT

Psychological preparation for a kidney transplant is mandatory for the recipient and their support network to overcome the psychological and emotional challenges posed by the procedure. This includes providing information and education about the transplant process, discussing the expected timetable, offering psychological assistance, teaching adaptive techniques like deep breathing, mindfulness and visualisation, setting reasonable expectations about the healing process, encouraging peer and social support through forums or support groups, also fostering open communication among family members.

Previous mental health disorders should be addressed and treated and mental health specialists should work together to provide appropriate care and support.

Short- and long-term objectives should be established to keep the patient motivated and purposeful during the healing process.

After transplant, it is essential to discuss the difficulties and modifications that may arise, such as continuing medical follow-ups, lifestyle changes and medication adherence. It is essential to stress the importance of asking for assistance and expressing concerns as soon as possible.

The transplant journey involves a continuous process of psychological preparation and a successful approach requires a multidisciplinary attitude including medical doctors, mental health specialists and the patient's support system.

By tailoring assistance to the specific needs of the transplant recipient and their support network, the process of psychological preparation for kidney transplantation can be made more manageable and successful.

POST-TRANSPLANT NUTRITION BASICS

It is important to eat a balanced, healthful diet after a kidney transplant in order to promote recuperation and preserve general wellbeing.

Here are some fundamentals of post-kidney transplant nutrition:

Hydration: Sufficient hydration is essential for renal health. Throughout the day, sip on plenty of water, but for advice on precise fluid consumption depending on your particular requirements, speak with your healthcare team.

Consumption of Protein: Protein is necessary for both repairing and preserving muscle mass. Lean protein sources including fish, chicken, eggs, dairy, tofu and lentils should all be a part of your diet. For individualised protein recommendations, nevertheless, speak with your healthcare team.

Limit Sodium *(Salt)* **Consumption:** Consuming too much salt will raise blood pressure, which can put stress on the kidneys. Steer clear of packaged and processed meals to reduce your sodium consumption, and consider seasoning food with herbs and spices rather than salt.

Control Potassium Levels: Because excessive potassium may be hazardous, patients of kidney transplants may need to watch how much potassium they eat. Bananas, oranges, tomatoes and potatoes are among the foods high in potassium. Assist your medical team in determining the right potassium intake for you.

Keep an eye on phosphorus levels since they may rise after a kidney transplant. Eat less high-phosphorus foods, such as nuts, dairy products and certain processed meals. You will get guidance on maintaining a good balance of phosphorus from your healthcare staff.

Calcium Intake: Healthy bones depend on getting enough calcium. Consume foods that are fortified with calcium, such as dairy products, leafy green vegetables and other meals. *If necessary*, your healthcare staff could suggest calcium supplements.

Consume Moderate Amounts of Fat: Opt for healthy fats like those in nuts, seeds, avocados, and olive oil. Reduce your intake of trans and saturated fats, since these may exacerbate cardiovascular problems.

Vitamin and Mineral Supplements: To promote general health, your medical staff may suggest vitamin and mineral supplements, such as vitamin D. Observe their recommendations when using supplements.

Reduce Your Sugar Intake: Eating a lot of sugar may lead to weight gain and other health problems. Limit additional sugars and choose for whole meals, especially in processed and sugary drinks.

Track Weight: Eat a balanced diet and engage in regular exercise to maintain a healthy weight. While severe weight loss may be an indication of starvation, rapid weight gain may be a symptom of fluid retention.

Customising your dietary plan to fit your unique requirements, medical history, and current medicines is essential.

CHAPTER 2: Dietary Restrictions and Recommendations

Post - Kidney Transplant

Following dietary recommendations is essential after a kidney transplant in order to support general health and guarantee the donated kidney functions properly. It's important to remember that exact recommendations could change depending on certain medical conditions, prescription drugs and the guidance of your healthcare team.

These are basic dietary guidelines and suggestions for those who have had a kidney transplant:

Fluid Consumption: The kidney that was transplanted may not be as good at regulating fluid intake, so pay close attention to how much you drink.
- Observe the guidance provided by your medical staff on daily fluid intake limits.

Intake of Sodium (Salt): Reduce your consumption of salt to assist control your blood pressure and lessen fluid retention.

- Steer clear of excess salt and opt for low-sodium or salt-free spices while preparing meals.

- Processed and packaged foods should be avoided since they often have high salt content.

Consumption of Protein: To maintain general health, keep your protein consumption moderate but not excessive.

- Select for lean meats, poultry, fish, eggs and dairy products as well as other high-quality protein sources.

- Speak with a dietician to find out how much protein you require on an individual basis.

Consumption of Potassium: Some people may need to restrict their consumption of potassium, particularly if their blood levels are high.

- Eat less high-potassium foods, such oranges, bananas, tomatoes, potatoes and certain legumes.

- Certain cooking techniques, such as boiling or soaking, may assist lower the potassium level of food.

Consumption of Phosphorus: Keep an eye on your phosphorus consumption, particularly if you have high blood phosphorus problems.

- Eat less of the foods high in phosphorus, such as dairy, nuts, seeds and carbonated drinks.

Consumption of Calcium: Continue to consume enough calcium to maintain healthy bones.

- Select calcium sources with low phosphorus content, such as leafy green vegetables, certain fruits and fortified cereals.

Limit Foods High in Purines: Reducing high-purine meals may be required for some persons in order to control their uric acid levels.

- Seafood, certain meats and organ meats are among the foods rich in purines.

Avoid Tobacco and Alcohol: Drinking alcohol may affect kidney function and interfere with drugs, so cut down or stay away from it.

- Give up smoking as it might harm your kidneys and your health in general.

Food Security: To lower the risk of infections—which may be more severe in those with weakened immune systems—practise appropriate food safety.

Frequent Inspections and Modifications: Keep a regular eye on your kidney function, blood pressure and other pertinent health indicators.

- In close collaboration with your medical team and a certified dietician, modify your diet as needed to suit your specific requirements.

FLUID INTAKE GUIDELINES

Remain Hydrated: Sustaining kidney function and general health requires consuming enough fluids. It keeps you from becoming dehydrated and promotes your replacement kidney's healthy operation.

Individualised Recommendations: Taking into account your age, weight, general health and kidney function, your healthcare team will provide recommendations on how much fluid you should drink.

Monitoring Fluid Balance: Your medical team may keep a careful eye on your fluid balance, which entails recording both your intake and excretion of fluids. By doing this, you can make sure that your equilibrium is stable and steer clear of issues like fluid retention or dehydration.

Limiting Some Beverages: Although it's crucial to keep hydrated, you could be told to cut down on or stay away from some drinks. For instance, it may not be advisable to consume large amounts of sugary or caffeinated beverages.

Electrolyte balance: It's critical to keep electrolytes like sodium and potassium in check. Your medical staff will advise you on how much and where to get these electrolytes in your diet.

Medication Consideration: Certain post-transplant drugs may have an impact on your fluid balance. It's important that you take your prescriptions as directed and let your medical team know if you have any adverse affects or concerns.

Keeping an Eye Out for Symptoms of Fluid Overload or Dehydration: Keep an eye out for symptoms of either condition, such as edema, elevated blood pressure or dark urine, dizziness or swelling. As soon as you notice any worrying signs, get in touch with your doctor.

Dietary Changes: You may need to make dietary changes to maintain the health of your kidneys. This might include limiting the amount of particular nutrients you consume, such as phosphorus, protein, and salt.

BUILDING A HEALTHY PLATE

After a kidney transplant, it is essential to maintain a healthy lifestyle and diet to support overall well-being and prevent complications. Here are general guidelines for building a healthy plate post-transplant:

1. A balanced diet involving a variety of foods from all food groups, including fruits, vegetables, grains, protein sources and dairy alternatives. A balanced distribution

of macronutrients, including carbohydrates, proteins and healthy fats.

2. Limit sodium intake to manage blood pressure and reduce fluid retention. Choose fresh, whole foods over processed and packaged ones, as they are lower in sodium.

3. Monitor fluid intake, as excessive fluid can strain the kidneys. Include foods with high water content, such as fruits and vegetables.

4. Choose lean protein sources like poultry, fish, tofu, and legumes.

5. Monitor phosphorus and potassium levels, adjusting intake based on healthcare provider's advice. Limit added sugars and opt for natural sources of sweetness like fruits.

6. Follow specific vitamin or mineral supplements, such as calcium or vitamin D, based on individual needs.

7. Practise good food safety, washing fruits and vegetables thoroughly, cooking meat thoroughly, and avoiding raw or undercooked seafood.

8. Regularly monitor weight, blood pressure, and laboratory values as advised by your healthcare team.

Communicate any changes in health or dietary habits with healthcare providers.

Maintaining a healthy lifestyle and diet post-transplant is mandatory for overall well-being and preventing complications.

CHAPTER 3: Portion Control and Meal Frequency

Meal frequency and portion management are essential components of post-transplant nutrition.

Here are some pointers to think about:

CONTROLLED PORTION

Well-Balanced Diet:

Prioritise eating a diet rich in a range of fruits, vegetables, whole grains, lean meats and healthy fats.

Reduce your consumption of added sweets, processed foods and saturated fats.

Consumption of Protein:

It's mandatory to consume enough protein for post-transplant recuperation. Incorporate lean protein sources into your meals, such as beans, fish, chicken and low-fat dairy.

To ascertain your individual protein requirements, speak with a dietician or your healthcare team.

Limitation of Sodium:

Limit your consumption of salt to help control blood pressure and lower your chance of developing fluid retention.

Steer clear of processed meals high in sodium and use as little salt as possible while preparing and serving.

Adaptable Administration:

In addition to avoiding excessive fluid retention, pay attention to your fluid intake to avoid dehydration.

If necessary, your healthcare provider will offer you instructions about your fluid limitations.

Mineral and vitamin supplements:

In order to address such deficiencies, take any vitamin and mineral supplements that have been given as directed by your healthcare provider.

FREQUENCY OF MEALS

Typical Meals:

For a consistent supply of nutrition and energy throughout the day, aim for frequent, well-balanced meals.

To keep your blood sugar levels consistent, try not to miss meals.

Snack Time:

Choose nutritious snacks like almonds, yoghurt, fresh fruits or vegetables if you are hungry in between meals.

Pay attention to serving amounts even while you're snacking.

When to Eat:

To ensure that you are getting enough nutrients throughout the day, space out your meals and snacks equally.

Observe any special recommendations for meal time that your healthcare provider may have given you.

Tracking Blood Sugar:

If you have diabetes, be sure to periodically check your blood sugar levels and modify your diet and snacks appropriately.

Tailored Strategy:

Create a personalised meal plan with the help of a certified dietician, taking into consideration your age, weight, exercise level and any other medical concerns.

Never forget how important it is to stay in contact with your healthcare team and to heed any dietary advice they may give you. Having regular check-ups with both your dietician and healthcare practitioner may assist guarantee that your dietary plan is modified as necessary according to your general health and healing process.

MEAL PLANNING FOR RECOVERY

The general diet guidelines highlight the importance of hydration, sodium control, protein intake and phosphorus and potassium levels.

Hydration is mandatory, especially water and sugary beverages should be limited.

Sodium control involves monitoring sodium intake, choosing fresh, whole foods and limiting table salt and high-sodium condiments.

Protein intake should include lean meats, poultry, fish, eggs, dairy and plant-based proteins.

Phosphorus and potassium levels should be monitored, with high-phosphorus foods like dairy and processed foods limited and potassium moderated.

Suggested Meals:

a. Muesli for breakfast, topped with berries and almonds.

toasted whole-grain bread with scrambled eggs with spinach.

Smoothie using low phosphorus fruits.

b. Lunch would be a salad of mixed veggies and olive oil dressing topped with grilled chicken or tofu.

Roasted veggie quinoa dish with a little amount of healthy protein.

Soup made with lentils and wholegrain crackers.

c. Fish baked or grilled with quinoa and steamed veggies for dinner.

Lean beef or tofu stir-fried with a rainbow of vibrant veggies.

Brown rice, low-potassium veggies on the side and grilled chicken.

d. Snacks: Berries or pieces of fresh fruit.

Greek yoghurt with a honey drizzle.

Hummus served with carrot or cucumber sticks.

Things to Think About:

a. ***Drug and Food Interactions:*** Pay attention to any interactions that may occur between your immunosuppressive drugs and certain meals. Seek advice from your healthcare team.

b. ***Customised Plan:*** Consult a certified dietitian to develop a meal plan that is tailored to your individual requirements, taking into account things like age, weight and any pre-existing medical issues.

c. ***Frequent Monitoring:*** As directed by your healthcare provider, monitor your blood pressure, weight and laboratory findings.

Safety Measures:

a. ***Food Safety:*** In light of the immunosuppressive drugs, observe appropriate food safety procedures to lower the risk of infection.

b. *Consultation:* Before making any big dietary changes, always get advice from your medical team or a certified dietitian.

CHAPTER 4: Understanding the Interaction Between Immunosuppressants and Diet

For those using immunosuppressive drugs, the relationship between food and immunosuppressive medicines must be taken into account.

Immunosuppressants are often used to reduce the function of the immune system, frequently in relation to organ transplantation or the management of autoimmune disorders. These drugs assist in treating autoimmune diseases by lowering inflammation and preventing the body from destroying newly donated organs or tissues.

The following are important things to think about when immunosuppressant and food interact:

Drug-Food Interactions: The absorption, metabolism, or efficacy of several immunosuppressants may be impacted by their interactions with specific foods. It's essential to adhere to the precise dietary recommendations made by chemists or medical specialists.

Interaction with Grapefruit: It is known that grapefruit juice and a number of drugs, including certain immunosuppressants, interact with each other. They have the ability to block the enzymes that are in charge of drug metabolism, which raises blood levels of the medication.

This may raise the possibility of toxicity or adverse consequences. When using immunosuppressants, people should ask their doctor about grapefruit interactions.

Vitamin and Mineral Deficiencies: The absorption of vitamins and minerals may be impacted by some immunosuppressants. For instance, the immunosuppressive drug corticosteroids may cause a decrease in bone density and calcium loss.

Long-term immunosuppressive treatment patients may need to keep an eye on their nutritional levels and take supplements as needed.

Drug-Nutrient Interactions: Certain nutrients and immunosuppressants may interact. *For example,* potassium levels may be impacted by cyclosporine, an immunosuppressant that is often administered. Medical professionals may check potassium levels and suggest dietary changes or supplementation as necessary.

Infection Risks: Immunosuppressants lessen the body's capacity to fight infections, increasing the risk of infection. Therefore, in order to reduce their risk of contracting foodborne infections, those using these drugs should adhere to the correct food safety recommendations.

This includes avoiding raw or undercooked food, maintaining proper cleanliness and using caution while handling foods that pose a danger.

Alcohol: It's important to talk about alcohol use with medical professionals since certain immunosuppressants may have unfavourable interactions with alcohol. Additionally, alcohol may have effects on the liver, which plays a role in the metabolism of drugs.

Weight management: Gaining weight or experiencing changes in body composition might result from some immunosuppressants. Nutritional measures to control weight and lower the risk of obesity-related problems may be suggested by healthcare professionals.

Healthcare experts, including physicians, chemists and nutritionists are the best people to ask for customised advice about immunosuppressive regimens and unique medical issues. They may provide advice on how to keep a balanced diet, deal with any medication interactions and take care of dietary issues.

TIMING MEALS AND MEDICATIONS

Post-kidney transplant care involves specific guidance from your medical team based on your health status, medications and recovery progress.

Immunosuppressive medications are crucial for maintaining proper drug levels and should be taken exactly as prescribed by your healthcare provider.

Meal timing is also essential, with many medications needing to be taken with food or on an empty stomach. Be aware of potential interactions between medications and certain foods, as some foods can affect the absorption of specific medications.

Fluid intake is important for managing kidney function and your healthcare team may provide guidelines on daily fluid intake.

Regular monitoring is essential, with follow-up appointments with your transplant team to adjust medications and address any concerns. If you have specific questions or concerns about meal timing and medications, consult your healthcare team for personalised advice based on your medical history and current condition.

It is important to remember that individual medical advice may vary and the information provided is not a substitute for professional healthcare guidance.

ADDRESSING COMMON CHALLENGES

Following a kidney transplant, the recovery period is vital and requires close monitoring of many areas of health and wellbeing. While every person's experience is unique, transplant recipients often encounter some difficulties throughout the post-kidney transplant recovery phase.

It's important to remember that the medical experts supervising the transplant should be consulted for specialised medical guidance.

The following are some common issues and ideas for solving them:

Drugs for Immunosuppression:

Challenge: Immunosuppressive drugs must be taken by transplant patients in order to avoid rejection, yet these drugs may cause adverse consequences.

Addressing: Take your medications according to the recommended regimen. Share any worries or side effects with the medical staff in an honest and transparent manner. Frequent blood tests assist in assessing medication levels and modifying doses as necessary.

Risk of Infection:

Problem: Immunosuppressive medications may make infections more likely.

Addressing: Maintain proper cleanliness, stay out of crowds during flu season, acquire the appropriate immunisations and notify the medical staff as soon as you see any symptoms of illness.

Monitoring Rejection:

Challenge: Rejection is a constant possibility that doesn't always show up as obvious symptoms.

Addressing: Make sure you show up for all planned follow-up sessions, have routine blood work done, and report any unexpected symptoms right away. Timely intervention is made possible by early discovery of rejection.

Discomfort and Pain after surgery:

Challenge: Following surgery, pain and suffering are frequent.

Addressing: Adhere to the recommended pain management regimen. Resuming physical activity gradually is encouraged by medical authorities. Inform the medical staff of any severe or ongoing discomfort.

Modifications to Diet:

Challenge: Restrictions and modifications to diet are often required.

Addressing: Adhere to the dietary guidelines that the transplant team recommends. Keep a healthy, balanced diet and observe the limits on your consumption of potassium, salt and fluids.

Balance of Fluids and Electrolytes:

Challenge: It might be difficult to maintain the proper ratio of electrolytes and water.

Resolving: As directed, keep an eye on your fluid intake and outflow. Observe the dietary recommendations for sodium and potassium. Inform the medical staff of any symptoms of electrolyte imbalance or dehydration.

Emotional Health:

Challenge: During the healing process, emotional difficulties like anxiety or despair might surface.

Addressing: Ask friends, relatives, or mental health specialists for help. Take part in transplant recipient support groups. Notify the medical staff of any serious emotional issues.

Practical and Financial Aspects to Take Into Account:

Challenge: The process of transplantation may be costly and logistically complex.

Addressing: Look into the financial aid options that are accessible. Speak with social workers and support groups to get advice on how to handle real-world difficulties.

Continuation Care:

Difficulty: Adhering strictly to follow-up treatment could be difficult.

Handling: Attend all of your visits on time, follow your doctor's advice on medication and lifestyle modifications and notify the medical staff of any issues as soon as possible.

Maintaining Long-Term Health:

Challenge: Preventing problems and preserving long-term health.

Managing: Adhere to the suggested lifestyle modifications, which include consistent physical activity, a well-rounded diet and abstaining from tobacco and excessive alcohol use. Learn about the significance of maintaining your health throughout time.

CHAPTER 5: Dealing with Taste Changes and Appetite Fluctuations

Post-kidney transplant recovery can lead to various body changes, including taste changes and appetite fluctuations. It is necessary to consult with your healthcare team for personalised advice.

Some general tips to manage these changes include staying hydrated, focusing on a balanced diet, experimenting with flavours, eating smaller frequent meals and incorporating lean protein sources like poultry, fish, eggs, dairy or plant-based alternatives.

A registered dietitian with experience in post-transplant nutrition can provide personalised advice to plan meals that meet nutritional needs and address taste changes. Monitor medication side effects and discuss any concerns with your transplant team to explore potential adjustments.

Gradually introduce new foods to your system and be patient with yourself to allow your taste buds to adapt. Regular physical activity can stimulate appetite and contribute to overall well-being.

Consult with your healthcare team to determine an appropriate exercise routine for your recovery.

Emotional support is essential as it plays a significant role in appetite and taste perception. Seek support from friends, family or a mental health professional if needed.

COPING WITH DIGESTIVE ISSUES

To manage digestive issues, it is essential to stay hydrated, eat a fibre-rich diet and consider incorporating probiotics.

Manage medications like immunosuppressants and antibiotics, as they can affect digestion. Monitor electrolyte levels and follow healthcare team recommendations for proper support.

Eat smaller, frequent meals to manage discomfort and promote overall well-being. Engage in regular, moderate physical activity to stimulate digestion and also limit processed foods and high-fat foods, focusing on a balanced diet.

Avoid trigger foods like spicy, acidic or high-fibre foods that may trigger discomfort. If digestive issues persist or worsen, consult your healthcare team for tailored advice and interventions. It is crucial to consult with your healthcare team before starting any new exercise regimen.

CHAPTER 6: Physical Activity and Wellness

INCORPORATING EXERCISE INTO THE RECOVERY ROUTINE

Exercise can enhance physical and mental well-being after a kidney transplant, but it's essential to consult with your healthcare team to ensure it aligns with your individual health status and recovery plan.

Start slowly with low-intensity exercises and gradually increase intensity as your body adjusts. Focus on cardiovascular exercise, such as walking, cycling or swimming to improve endurance and energy levels.

Incorporate light resistance training, using light weights and performing a higher number of repetitions.

Incorporate flexibility exercises to improve range of motion and reduce stiffness, especially if you have post-surgery limitations in movement.

Pay attention to your body's response to exercise and stop if you experience pain, discomfort or unusual symptoms. Stay well-hydrated by drinking water before, during and after exercise. Monitor vital signs like heart rate, blood pressure and other vital signs while exercising to assess your response to physical activity.

Schedule regular check-ups with your healthcare team to discuss progress, address concerns and make adjustments to your exercise routine if necessary. Mind-body exercises, such as meditation, deep breathing exercises or tai chi, can support mental well-being and complement physical activity.

Remember that every individual is unique and the post-transplant recovery process varies.

STRESS MANAGEMENT STRATEGIES

For those who have had a kidney transplant, stress management is essential as it may improve general health and increase the likelihood that the transplant will be successful.

These techniques might be useful for stress management in kidney transplant recipients:

Meditation with Mindfulness:

To help you relax, concentrate on the here and now, and manage anxiety, try mindfulness meditation. Apps for mindfulness or guided meditation sessions might be used for this.

Breathing Techniques:

Include deep breathing techniques in your everyday practice to assist lower stress and soothe the neurological system. Breathing deeply and slowly might help you relax and feel better mentally overall.

Exercise:

Follow your healthcare team's recommendations and exercise regularly but moderately. Exercise produces endorphins, which have been shown to lessen stress and enhance happiness. Be sure to speak with your doctor before beginning a new fitness programme.

Support Teams:
Become a member of a transplant recipient support group. Emotional support and coping mechanisms

may be obtained by sharing emotions and experiences with others who have experienced comparable circumstances.

Therapeutic Methods:

If you're having emotional difficulties, worry or stress, think about using therapeutic methods like cognitive-behavioural therapy (CBT) or counselling.

Methods of Relaxation:

To ease tension and stress, try relaxation methods like progressive muscle relaxation, biofeedback or guided visualisation.

Choosing a Healthier Lifestyle:

Keep yourself healthy by eating a well-balanced diet, drinking enough water, getting enough sleep and limiting your intake of alcohol and caffeine.

Effective Time Management:

Set priorities for your work and practise good time management to lessen overload. Divide up the work into smaller, easier-to-complete segments.

Communicate Yourself:

Talk to a mental health professional, trustworthy family members, or friends about your emotions and concerns. Emotional burdens may be lessened and important assistance can be given with open communication.

Calming Activities:

Take part in enjoyable and soothing activities, such reading, listening to music, taking in the outdoors, or taking up a hobby.

Learn for Yourself:

Find out more about your transplant and the care that comes after. Gaining knowledge may give you confidence and allay worries, which can help you feel in control and less stressed.

Sustain an Optimistic attitude:

Develop an optimistic outlook by concentrating on the things in your life that make you happy and grateful. Celebrate your recovery's little accomplishments and significant milestones.

CHAPTER 7: Adapting Nutritional Habits for Sustainable Health

Greetings on your successful kidney transplant! You must modify your eating habits if you want to stay healthy after a transplant.

These are some broad recommendations, but it's recommended to speak with your healthcare team for customised guidance according to your particular medical condition:

Kidney transplant patients should maintain proper hydration, protein intake, sodium intake, potassium levels, phosphorus and calcium intake, blood sugar levels and weight management.

They should drink plenty of water, consume enough protein for muscle mass maintenance and repair, and also limit sodium intake to control blood pressure and fluid retention.

Potassium is crucial for bone health, phosphorus and calcium should be balanced through fortified meals, leafy greens and dairy products.

Regular monitoring is essential due to potential transplant drug effects on these levels. Phosphorus consumption can be restricted in kidney-friendly diets, such as avoiding processed foods and chocolate.

Maintaining a healthy weight is essential for general health and can reduce the risk of diabetes and hypertension. Food safety is crucial and healthcare staff may suggest supplements like vitamin D or iron based on individual needs and test findings.

Periodic Nutritional Assessments and Adjustments

A nutritious, well-balanced diet is Important for the recipient's general health after a kidney transplant. In addition to addressing any unique demands or difficulties associated with the transplant, nutritional evaluations and modifications are critical to guaranteeing that the body gets the nutrients it requires.

Regarding dietary therapy after a kidney transplant, keep the following in mind:

Consumption of Protein:

Sufficient protein is necessary for immunological response and tissue repair. Nonetheless, consuming too much protein might further tax the kidneys. A nutritionist can assist in figuring out how much protein is acceptable depending on renal function and personal requirements.

Flowing Equilibrium:

Proper hydration is mandatory, but excessive fluid consumption may lead to concerns like hypertension or fluid retention. It's critical to keep an eye on fluid balance, particularly for those with impaired kidney function. Seek advice from a medical expert to determine the right amount of fluid consumption.

Intake of Sodium (Salt):

Controlling salt consumption aids in maintaining fluid balance and blood pressure. In order to avoid hypertension and fluid retention, recipients of transplants are often recommended to restrict their salt consumption. Eat fresh, unprocessed foods whenever possible since processed foods and restaurant meals might have excessive salt content. Make sure you read labels carefully.

Potassium and Calcium:

Patients receiving transplants may be more susceptible to problems with their bones as a result of drugs and altered mineral metabolism. Monitoring calcium and phosphorus levels is important and a medical expert may suggest dietary changes or supplementation.

Minerals and Vitamins:

Certain vitamins and minerals may not be absorbed as well when taken with immunosuppressive drugs. It's critical to regularly check nutritional levels, particularly those of vitamin D and B vitamins. In the event that inadequacies are found, supplements could be recommended.

Consumption of Calories:

Sustaining a healthy weight is critical to general health. Underweight people may need to consume more calories, while overweight people might need to concentrate on managing their weight. A dietitian's customised guidance is crucial.

Nutritional Limitations:

Dietary restrictions may be necessary for some drugs and medical conditions. *For instance*, it's usually advised to stay away from grapefruit and grapefruit juice because of possible interactions with immunosuppressive medications.

Frequent Observation:

It is important to schedule routine follow-up visits with a dietician, nephrologist and transplant team in order to assess nutritional status and make necessary modifications. To evaluate renal function and nutritional levels, blood tests may be performed.

Customised Method:

The dietary requirements of transplant patients might differ. Making a customised nutrition plan requires an individualised strategy that considers things like age, gender, exercise level and medical history.

A qualified dietitian and other members of the transplant recipient's healthcare team should collaborate closely to create and modify a dietary plan that suits their individual requirements and promotes general health after kidney transplantation.

NEXT PAGE:

20 Nutrient-Rich Recipes

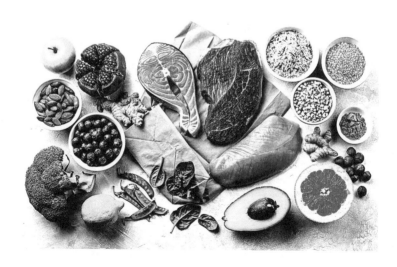

20 POST KIDNEY TRANSPLANT RECIPES THAT HELPS DURING YOUR HEALING PROCESS.

BREAKFAST

Vegetable Omelette:

Ingredients:

- three eggs
- 1/4 cup of chopped red, green, or yellow bell peppers
- one-fourth cup of chopped tomatoes
- one-fourth cup of finely chopped onions
- 1/4 cup finely chopped kale or spinach
- To taste, add salt and pepper.
- One tablespoon of butter or olive oil
- Shredded cheese *(your choice of mozzarella, cheddar or both)* is optional.

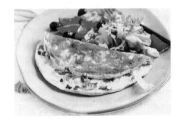

Instructions:

Get the veggies ready:
Chop the onions, tomatoes and bell peppers.
Chop the spinach or kale.

Beat the Eggs:
Place the cracked eggs in a basin.
Using a fork or whisk, thoroughly combine the eggs.

Spiced Eggs:
Toss in the beaten eggs along with a touch of salt and pepper. You may change the seasoning to suit your preferences.

Sautéed Vegetables:
In a nonstick skillet, preheat the butter or olive oil over medium heat.

Add the chopped onions and cook them until they are transparent.

After adding the bell peppers, sauté them until they start to become soft.

When the tomatoes start to release their juices, simmer them for a few more minutes.
Finally, add chopped spinach or kale and simmer until wilted.

Transfer Eggs:
Over the pan with sautéed veggies, pour the beaten eggs.

Cook and Swirl:
After giving the eggs a minute to set, carefully rotate the pan to make sure everything cooks evenly.

Using a spatula, gently raise the edges as they harden to allow the raw eggs to flow below.

Cheese Addition (Optional):

If you prefer, add shredded cheese over one side of the omelette.

Fold the omelette in half using a spatula after the eggs are set but still somewhat wet on top.
Slide the omelette onto a plate and serve while hot.

Optional garnish:
For extra flavour, garnish with fresh herbs like chives or parsley.

Low-fat Greek yoghourt with fresh berries and a sprinkle of nuts Smoothie Bowl:

Ingredients:

- 1 cup Greek yoghurt with reduced fat
- 1/2 cup of fresh berries *(a combination of raspberries, blueberries and strawberries)*
- One-fourth cup granola
- Two teaspoons of finely chopped nuts *(you may use walnuts or almonds)*.
- One tablespoon of maple syrup or honey *(optional; adds sweetness)*
- Garnish with fresh mint leaves *(optional)*.

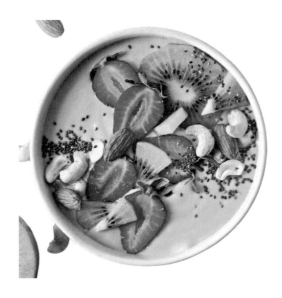

Instruction:

In a blender, mix the low-fat Greek yoghurt with half of the fresh berries. Process till smooth.

Transfer the berry mixture and yoghurt into a bowl.

Over the smoothie base, distribute the remaining fresh berries, granola and chopped almonds.

Drizzle some honey or maple syrup on top for a sweeter flavour.

Add some fresh mint leaves as a garnish for visual appeal and a refreshing touch.

Savour your mouth watering smoothie bowl right away, when the components are still fresh and the texture is flawless.

You are welcome to alter the recipe to suit your tastes. You may boost the nutritious content by adding additional fruits, flaxseeds or chia seeds. Not only is this smoothie bowl delicious, but it also has a sensible ratio of fibre, protein and healthy fats to keep you full and focused all day.

Whole Grain Pancakes

Ingredients:

- One cup of flour *made from whole wheat*
- One spoonful of sugar
- One tsp baking powder
- One-half tsp baking soda
- 1/4 tsp salt
- 1 cup of buttermilk
- One big egg
- Two teaspoons of vegetable oil or melted butter
- *Optional:* One tsp vanilla essence
- *Optional:* Half a cup of chopped nuts or blueberries

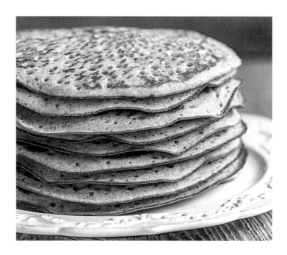

Instruction:

Mix the whole wheat flour, sugar, baking soda, baking powder and salt in a large mixing dish.

Whisk the buttermilk, egg, melted butter or oil and vanilla extract *(if using)* in another basin.

Stirring gently until well mixed then pour the wet components into the dry ingredients.

Take care not to overmix; some lumps are OK.

Add chopped nuts or blueberries, *if preferred*, and fold gently.

Heat a nonstick skillet or griddle to medium. Apply a tiny quantity of butter or cooking spray to the surface to lightly oil it.

For each pancake - place 1/4 cup amounts of batter onto the griddle. Cook until surface bubbles appear, then turn and continue cooking until golden brown on the other side.

Continue until all of the batter has been used, reheating the fried pancakes in a low oven *if needed*.

Top the whole grain pancakes with your preferred ingredients, such yoghurt, fresh fruit, maple syrup or chopped nuts. Serve.

Quinoa Breakfast Bowl

Ingredients:

- One cup of washed quinoa
- Two cups of almond milk or any other kind of milk you like.
- One tsp vanilla essence
- One tablespoon of maple syrup, *if desired*
- One cup of mixed berries, including raspberries, blueberries and strawberries.
- 1/4 cup chopped nuts *(almonds, walnuts or pecans)*
- one sliced banana
- Two tsp of chia seeds
- Greek yoghurt is *optional.*
- Drizzling honey *(optional)*

Instruction:

Rinse the quinoa and put it in a medium pot with almond milk. After bringing to a boil, lower the heat to a simmer then cover and let the quinoa cook for about 15 minutes or until the liquid has been absorbed.

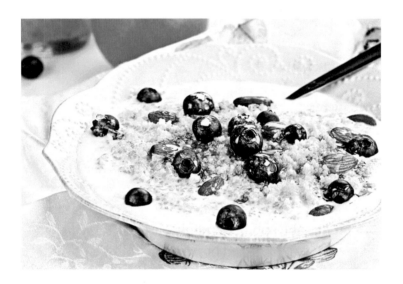

If using, stir in the maple syrup and vanilla extract. While the quinoa is cooking, prepare your toppings. Clean and cut the banana and berries then cut the nuts into pieces.

Spoon cooked quinoa into each of the serving dishes.

Add chopped almonds, chia seeds, banana slices and mixed berries to the top of each bowl.

Extras that are optional:

For a creamy finish, top with a dollop of Greek yoghurt or pour some honey over it for more sweetness.

While still warm, serve the quinoa breakfast dish right away.

You can alter this recipe to suit your tastes. You may experiment with other nuts or seeds and add other fruits, like mango or kiwi. This breakfast bowl is loaded with fibre, protein and other vital nutrients to help you get off to a healthy start.

Egg and Spinach Breakfast Wrap

Ingredients:

- Two big eggs
- One cup of freshly cleaned and cut Spinach leaves
- One tablespoon of olive oil
- *To taste,* Salt and pepper.
- One tortilla with spinach or whole wheat flavour
- *Add-ons:* Sliced avocado, salsa and shredded cheese

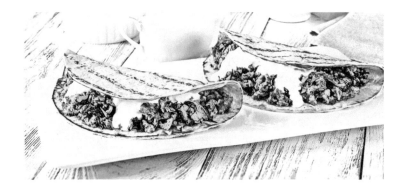

Instruction:

One tablespoon of olive oil is heated over medium heat in a skillet.

Sauté the chopped spinach in the pan for two to three minutes or until it wilts.

To taste, add salt and pepper for seasoning. Put aside.

Crack two eggs into the same pan and cook till desired *(scrambled, fried or poached)*.
Add salt and pepper to the eggs for seasoning.
To make the tortilla malleable, warm it for approximately 10 seconds in a pan or microwave.

Arrange the cooked spinach in a layer in the centre of the tortilla on a level surface.

Place the scrambled eggs over the spinach.

While the eggs are still warm, cover them with shredded cheese and let them melt a little bit.

Add avocado slices for smoothness and salsa for a taste explosion.

To cover the eggs and toppings, fold the tortilla's edges towards the centre.

Keeping the bottom of the wrap securely rolled, create a tidy little package.

If desired, cut the wrap in half diagonally to make it simpler to handle.

Enjoy your wholesome egg and spinach breakfast wrap right away after serving.

Alter the recipe by using additional items you like, including black beans, chopped tomatoes, or a splash of spicy sauce.

LUNCH

Grilled Chicken Salad

Ingredients:

The Chicken Grilled:
- Two skinless and boneless chicken breasts
- Two tsp olive oil
- one tsp powdered garlic
- One tsp of paprika
- *To taste*, add salt and pepper.

For the Salad:
- Mixed greens for salad *(arugula, lettuce, spinach, etc.)*
- *For the dressing* - Chop cherry tomatoes, cut cucumber in half, slice red bell pepper, slice red onion and thinly slice avocado.

- Turmeric
- 3 Tablespoons of extra virgin
- Half a tsp balsamic vinegar
- One tsp Dijon mustard
- 1 minced garlic clove
- *To taste*, add salt and pepper.

Instructions:

To make a marinade, combine olive oil, salt, pepper, paprika and garlic powder in a basin.

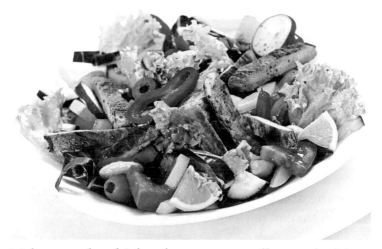

Make sure the chicken breasts are well coated with the marinade.

Place it in the fridge to marinate for at least half an hour.

Set the grill's temperature to medium-high.
The chicken should be cooked through after 6 to 8 minutes on each side of the grill.

A temperature of 165°F (74°C) should be reached inside.

After cooking, let the chicken rest for a few minutes before slicing it into thin pieces.

The avocado, cherry tomatoes, cucumber, red bell pepper, red onion and mixed salad greens should all be combined in a big bowl.

Preparing the Dressing:

Mix the olive oil, balsamic vinegar, Dijon mustard, minced garlic, salt and pepper in a small bowl until well blended.

Pour the dressing over the salad and gently toss to ensure that all of the items are coated.

Arrange the grilled chicken pieces over the salad and serve right away after dividing it among plates.

Salmon Wrap

Ingredients:

- Two fillets of salmon
- *To taste*, Salt and pepper.
- One tablespoon of olive oil
- 4 wraps, whole wheat or spinach

- half a cup of Greek yoghurt
- Mayonnaise, 2 tablespoons
- One spoonful of mustard dijon
- one tsp lemon juice
- One tsp honey
- Two cups of baby spinach leaves
- One cucumber, cut thinly
- One sliced avocado
- Half a red onion, cut thinly
- *For garnish,* use fresh dill *(optional).*

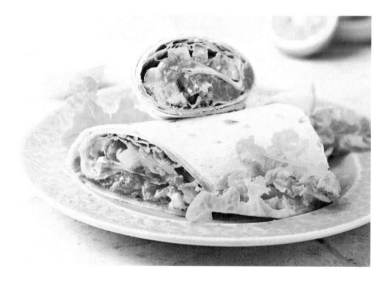

Instruction:

Set oven temperature to 400°F, or 200°C.

Use salt and pepper to season the salmon fillets. Heat olive oil in a pan over medium-high heat.

Sear the salmon fillets until golden brown, about 2 to 3 minutes each side.

When the salmon flakes easily with a fork and is cooked through, roughly 8 to 10 minutes should have passed, transfer it to the preheated oven.

For the sauce - Combine Greek yoghurt, lemon juice, honey, mayonnaise and Dijon mustard in a small bowl. Taste and adjust the seasoning.

To make the wraps more malleable, quickly reheat them in a dry pan in the microwave for 10 seconds.

Take a big dollop of the sauce and spread it on each wrap.

Divide the cooked salmon equally among the wraps by flaking it into bite-sized pieces.

Arrange the baby spinach leaves, cucumber, avocado and red onion slices in layers on the wraps.

For additional flavour, sprinkle some fresh dill over the fillings and drizzle a little more sauce over them.

To create a secure wrap, fold the sides of the wraps and roll them securely from the bottom.

Serve the wraps right away after cutting them in half diagonally.

Vegetable Stir-Fry

Ingredients:

- Two cups chopped mixed veggies *(broccoli, mushrooms, bell peppers, carrots, snap peas, etc.)*
- two tsp of vegetable oil
- 3 minced garlic cloves
- one tablespoon finely chopped ginger
- 1 spoonful of soy sauce
- 1 tablespoon of *optional,* Oyster sauce
- One tsp of sesame oil
- One teaspoon cornflour *(optional; used to make the sauce thicker)*
- *To taste,* Salt and Pepper.
- *Optional* Red pepper flakes for extra spiciness
- 2 sliced green onions *(for garnish)*
- Ready-to-serve cooked rice or noodles

Instruction:

Clean the veggies and cut them into little pieces.

Combine the cornflour, sesame oil, oyster sauce *(if using)*, and soy sauce in a small bowl. Put aside.

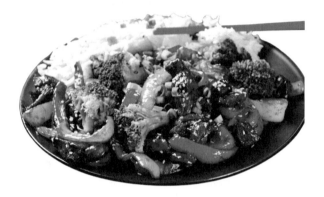

In a large pan or wok, heat the vegetable oil over medium-high heat.

Add the ginger and garlic, minced and sauté for 30 seconds or more - until fragrant.

First, add the tougher veggies *(broccoli and carrots)*, and stir-fry for two to three minutes or until the vegetables begin to soften.

After adding the other veggies, stir-fry them for a further 2 to 3 minutes, until they are all crisp-tender.

When you're done preparing the sauce, pour it over the veggies and toss to cover them evenly. Cook for an additional 1-2 minutes.

If preferred, add red pepper flakes, salt and pepper for seasoning. Garnish with chopped green onions.

Serve the veggie stir-fry over cooked rice or noodles.

Feel free to alter this dish by substituting your preferred protein—for example, prawns, chicken or tofu—into it. To suit your tastes, adjust the amount of sauce and spice.

Turkey and Avocado Sandwich

Ingredients:

- Turkey breast slices
- Sliced whole-grain bread or *the bread of your choice*
- Slices of 1 ripe avocado
- Lettuce stems
- Slabbed tomato
- Finely chopped red onion *(optional)*
- Mayonnaise
- Mustard
- *To taste*, Salt and pepper.

Instruction:

Slice and wash the red onion, avocado, and tomato. The lettuce leaves should be cleaned and pat dried.

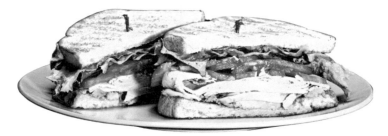

To add more flavour and texture, you may toast the bread pieces if you'd like.

Spread your preferred amount of mayonnaise and mustard on one side of each piece of bread.

Start by arranging one piece of bread with the turkey slices on it.
Arrange a layer of sliced avocado over the turkey.

Spoon over the avocado with the lettuce leaves.
If using, add the red onion and tomato slices.
To taste, add salt and pepper for seasoning.

To finish the sandwich, place the second piece of bread on top, condiment side down.

Cut the sandwich in half, *if you'd like*, carefully and diagonally.

Optional Add-ons:

You may add cheese, bacon or any other preferred toppings to personalise your sandwich. Think of using a variety of breads, including baguettes, sourdough or whole wheat.

You may finally savour your turkey and avocado sandwich. Serve it with a simple green salad or your favourite side dishes.

Quinoa and Black Bean Bowl

Ingredients:

- One cup of washed quinoa
- two cups of water
- One can *(15 oz)* of rinsed and drained black beans
- One cup of fresh or frozen corn kernels
- One sliced bell pepper, whichever colour you like
- Half a cup of cherry tomatoes

- One sliced avocado
- 1/4 cup of coarsely chopped red onion
- 1/4 cup finely chopped fresh cilantro
- one lime's juice
- Two tsp olive oil
- *To taste*, Salt and pepper.
- Salsa, sour cream and shredded cheese - *Optional garnishes.*

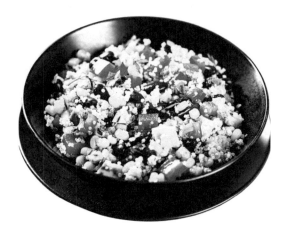

Instruction:

Quinoa and water should be combined in a medium pot. After bringing to a boil, lower the heat to a simmer and cover.

Let the quinoa cook for around fifteen minutes, or until the water has been absorbed. Once the quinoa is fluffy, let it cool.

Black beans, corn, chopped red pepper, cherry tomatoes, red onion and cilantro should all be combined in a big bowl.

Mix the lime juice, olive oil, salt and pepper in a small bowl.

Toss the chilled quinoa into the big dish of vegetables.

Over the quinoa and veggies, drizzle the lime dressing. Mix everything until well incorporated.

Spoon the black bean and quinoa mixture into individual serving dishes.

Add sliced avocado and any other desired toppings to the top of each bowl.

Serve the Quinoa and Black Bean Bowls right away.

You are welcome to alter this recipe to suit your tastes. For more protein, you may add tofu, grilled chicken or any other preferred protein.

DINNER

Baked Cod with Lemon

Ingredients:

- Four 6 ounce-per-fillet fish fillets
- Two tsp olive oil
- 2 tsp freshly squeezed lemon juice
- 2 minced garlic cloves
- One tsp of dehydrated oregano
- A single tsp of dried thyme
- 1 tsp of paprika
- *To taste*, Salt and pepper.
- Slices of lemon as a garnish
- Chop some fresh parsley for garnish.

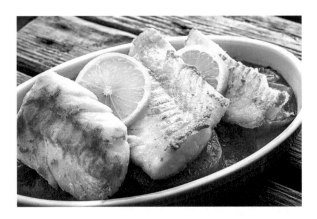

Instruction:

Set oven temperature to 400°F, or 200°C.

Grease a baking sheet gently or line it with parchment paper.

With some space between each fillet, place the cod fillets on the baking sheet that has been prepared.

Mix the olive oil, lemon juice, minced garlic, paprika, dried thyme, dried oregano, salt and pepper in a small bowl.

Make sure each fish fillet is well covered by brushing the mixture over the top of them.

For extra flavour, top each fillet with one or two slices of lemon.

Bake the fish for 15 to 20 minutes in a preheated oven or until it is opaque and flakes readily with a fork.

Take the cod out of the oven when it is cooked through.
If preferred, garnish with extra lemon slices and fresh parsley.

Serve the baked cod with your preferred side dishes, such rice, salad or steamed veggies.

Vegetable and Lentil Stew

Ingredients:

- One cup of dried, rinsed and drained Green or Brown lentils.
- 2 tsp olive oil
- 1 big onion, finely sliced
- 3 minced garlic cloves
- Two chopped and peeled carrots
- Two chopped celery stalks and one sliced bell pepper *(any colour)*
- One sliced zucchini and one can *(14 oz)* chopped Undrained tomatoes
- 4 cups of broth made with vegetables
- One tsp of dried oregano and one tsp of dried thyme
- One teaspoon of cumin powder
- One-half tsp smoked paprika
- *To taste*, Salt and pepper.
- 2 cups finely chopped kale or spinach
- One lemon, juiced *(optional for extra brightness)*

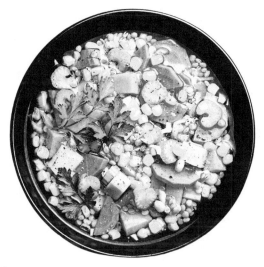

Instruction:

Heat the olive oil in a big saucepan over medium heat. Add the chopped onion and garlic and sauté.

Stir in the bell pepper, zucchini, celery and carrots. Cook, stirring regularly, until the veggies start to soften, approximately 5 minutes.

Add the lentils, thyme, cumin, oregano, chopped tomatoes *(with their juice)*, vegetable broth, smoky paprika, salt and pepper.

After bringing the stew to a boil, lower the heat to a simmer, cover it and let it cook for 25 to 30 minutes or until the lentils are soft.

Stir the chopped kale or spinach into the saucepan until it wilts.

If preferred, add a squeeze of lemon juice to the stew to give it a zesty boost.

Serve the hot lentil and vegetable stew after adjusting the spice.

If desired, you may top it with grated Parmesan cheese or a dollop of yoghurt along with fresh herbs like cilantro or parsley.

Sweet Potato and Chickpea Curry

Ingredients:

- Peel and dice two medium-sized sweet potatoes.
- One can *(15 oz)* of rinsed and drained chickpeas
- 1 onion, chopped finely
- 2 minced garlic cloves
- One tablespoon of grated ginger
- One 14-oz can of chopped tomatoes
- 1 can, or 14 ounces milk from coconuts
- 1 cup of veggie broth
- 2 teaspoons of curry powder

- One tsp ground coriander
- 1 tsp ground cumin
- 1/2 a teaspoon of turmeric
- Half a teaspoon of paprika
- *To taste,* Salt and pepper.
- 2 tsp of vegetable oil
- Finely chopped fresh cilantro *(for garnish)*
- Naan or cooked rice *(for serving)*

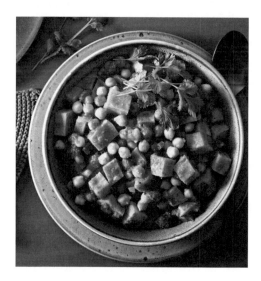

Instructions:

In a big saucepan or Dutch oven, heat the vegetable oil over medium heat. When the oil is hot, add the chopped onions and simmer till transparent.

Add the grated ginger and minced garlic and sauté for an additional 1 to 2 minutes or until aromatic.

To the saucepan, add the curry powder, paprika, turmeric, ground coriander and cumin. Stir vigorously to evenly distribute the spices over the onions, garlic and ginger.

When the sweet potatoes start to soften, add the diced ones to the saucepan and simmer, stirring bit by bit for 5 to 7 minutes.

Add the veggie broth, coconut milk and chopped tomatoes then simmer the mixture for a while.

Fill the saucepan with the rinsed and drained chickpeas.

To taste, add salt and pepper for seasoning.

Once the sweet potatoes are soft, around 20 to 25 minutes of medium-low heat or simmering time is required for the curry.

If necessary, taste and adjust the seasoning.
Serve the curry of sweet potatoes and chickpeas over naan or over cooked rice. Add freshly chopped cilantro as a garnish.

Grilled Shrimp Skewers

Ingredients:

- One pound of big, peeled and deveined prawns
- 2 tsp olive oil
- 3 minced garlic cloves
- One tsp of smoky paprika
- One teaspoon of cumin
- One tsp of chilli powder
- Half a teaspoon cayenne, *or more* - according to taste
- *To taste*, Salt and pepper.
- One lemon's juice
- Metal or wood skewers

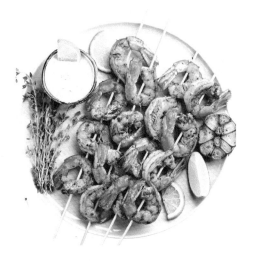

Instructions:

To keep wooden skewers from burning when grilling, immerse them in water for around half an hour.

Dry the shrimp by patting it with a paper towel.

Prepare the prawns by marinating them -

Olive oil, minced garlic, cumin, smoked paprika, chilli powder, cayenne pepper, salt and pepper should all be combined in a bowl.

Toss the prawns in the marinade to ensure uniform coating.

Give it a minimum of 15 to 20 minutes to marinade so the flavours can fully meld.

Make sure the skewer goes through each shrimp's body and tail as you thread the marinated shrimp onto the skewers.

Set your grill's temperature to medium-high.

The prawn skewers should be placed on the heating grill. Sear the prawns for 2 to 3 minutes on each side or until they become opaque and have a hint of char.

While the prawns are cooking, baste them with the leftover marinade.

Squeeze fresh lemon juice over the grilled prawns before serving.

Optional Garnish:
For a pop of freshness, add some chopped cilantro or parsley as a garnish.

Prepare a simple dipping sauce by blending extra virgin olive oil, minced garlic, lemon juice, salt and pepper.

These prawn skewers can be a delicious appetiser or main dish. For a satisfying and delectable dinner, pair them with your preferred side dishes, such grilled veggies or a salad.

Chicken and Vegetable Kebabs

Ingredients:

Regarding the Marinade:

- One pound *(450 grammes)* of skinless, boneless chicken breasts, diced into bite-sized pieces
- One-fourth cup of plain yoghurt
- Two tsp olive oil
- two tsp lemon juice

- 2 tsp finely chopped garlic
- One teaspoon of cumin powder
- One tsp of paprika
- One tsp finely ground coriander
- One tsp of turmeric
- *To taste*, Salt and pepper.

Regarding the Kebabs:

- Cut bell peppers into bits; for visual interest, *use a variety of colours.*
- Cut up red onion into pieces
- Rosy tomatoes
- Cut the zucchini into rounds.
- Metal or wood skewers

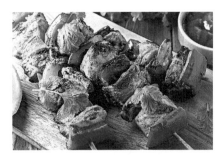

Instructions:

Combine the yoghurt, olive oil, lemon juice, minced garlic, cumin, paprika, coriander, turmeric, salt and pepper in a bowl to form the marinade.

Make sure all of the chicken cubes are properly coated before adding them to the marinade.

To enable the flavours to blend, cover the bowl and refrigerate for at least 30 minutes.

To keep wooden skewers from burning when grilling, immerse them in water for around half an hour.

Preheat your grill or oven to medium-high heat.

Alternating between the marinated chicken and the veggies,
thread the red peppers, red onion, cherry tomatoes and zucchini onto the skewers.

Put the kebabs in the oven or on the prepared grill.

Grill, rotating periodically for 12 to 15 minutes or until the chicken is cooked through and the veggies are soft and gently browned.

Before serving, take the kebabs out of the oven or grill and let them rest for a few minutes.

Serve the Chicken and Vegetable Kebabs with a squeeze of fresh lemon or your favourite sauce, such tzatziki or barbecue sauce.

SNACKS

Fruit Salad

Ingredients:

- Two cups of hulled and sliced strawberries
- One cup of blueberries
- One cup of halved grapes
- Two peeled and sliced kiwi fruits
- 1 peeled, pitted and chopped mango
- One sliced banana
- One peeled and segments orange

Regarding the Dressing:

- 2 tsp honey
- One tablespoon of freshly squeezed lime juice
- One teaspoon of optional poppy seeds

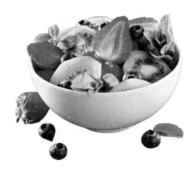

Instructions:

Combine all the prepared fruits in a big basin.

To prepare the dressing, combine the lime juice and honey in a small basin.

You may add poppy seeds for more flavour if you'd like.

After adding the dressing, carefully toss the fruit to ensure uniform coating.

To enable the flavours to mingle, place the fruit salad in the refrigerator for at least half an hour before serving.

Toss the fruit salad gently one again just before serving.

Hummus with Veggies

Ingredients:

- One can *(15 ounces)* of washed and drained garbanzo beans, or chickpeas
- 1 big lemon or 1/4 cup of fresh lemon juice

- 1/4 cup tahini, well mixed
- One little clove of chopped garlic
- 2 tablespoons of extra virgin olive oil, plus more to dress.
- half a teaspoon of cumin powder
- Salt to taste.
- 2 to 3 tsp water
- A pinch of paprika, *optional*, for serving

Veggie Dippers Ingredients:

- carrot sticks
- Slices of cucumber
- Strips of bell pepper, either green, yellow or red
- Rosy tomatoes
- florets of broccoli

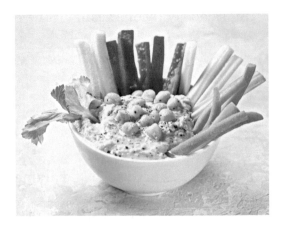

Instructions:

Add the chickpeas, olive oil, tahini, cumin, garlic and a dash of salt to a food processor.

Blend the ingredients until they are smooth. To make sure all the ingredients are well mixed, scrape down the sides of the bowl as necessary.

Add 2 to 3 tablespoons of water at a time while the food processor is running, until the hummus has the consistency you want.

Blend until smooth.

After tasting the hummus, adjust the spices by adding extra lemon juice or salt as necessary.

Move the hummus into a dish for serving. If you'd like, garnish with a pinch of paprika and a drizzle of olive oil.

Place the cut vegetables around the hummus on a dish for serving.

Present the hummus beside the mixed vegetables for dunkling.

Go ahead and use your imagination while choosing your vegetables. For extra flavour, you may also add chopped fresh herbs like cilantro or parsley.

Nuts and Seeds Mix

Ingredients:

- One cup of almonds
- One cup of walnuts
- One cup cashews
- half a cup of pumpkin seeds
- half a cup of sunflower seeds
- Half a cup of chia seeds
- half a cup of flax seeds
- 1/2 cup *(optional)* unsweetened coconut flakes
- Two teaspoons of honey or maple syrup
- One tablespoon of olive or coconut oil
- one tsp finely ground cinnamon
- half a teaspoon of sea salt

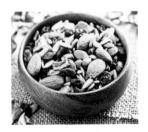

Instruction:

Set the oven temperature to 325°F (163°C).

Almonds, walnuts, cashews, pumpkin, sunflower, chia, flax and coconut flakes should all be combined in a big mixing basin.

Melt the coconut oil *(or olive oil)* in a small saucepan over low heat. Add maple syrup *(or honey)*, ground cinnamon and sea salt. Mix well until fully covered.

Over the nuts and seeds in the dish, pour the liquid mixture. Then toss to provide a uniform coating.

Evenly distribute the ingredients onto a parchment paper-lined baking sheet.

Bake for 15 to 20 minutes or until the nuts and seeds are golden brown, in a preheated oven.

To avoid burning, be careful to stir the mixture every five minutes.

Take it out of the oven and allow it to cool fully.

After the mixture of nuts and seeds has cooled, store it in an airtight container.

Customise the recipe by adding your favourite nuts or seeds, altering the sweetness or introducing additional spices like nutmeg or vanilla extract. You can add this mix to salads, oats or yoghurt for an added crunch. It also makes a fantastic snack on its own.

Greek Yoghurt with Honey

Ingredients:

- 2 Cups Greek yoghurt
- Two to three teaspoons of honey, taste-adjusting
- Fresh fruit (*chopped peaches, sliced bananas, or berries, for example*) - **optional Nuts** (*such chopped walnuts or almonds*) Leaves of mint for garnish - *Optional.*

Instruction:

You may strain normal yoghurt to produce your own Greek yoghurt if you don't have any in the shop.

After covering a bowl with a fresh kitchen towel or cheesecloth and adding the yoghurt, strain it in the fridge for several hours or overnight until the required thickness is achieved.

Transfer the Greek yoghurt into dishes for serving.

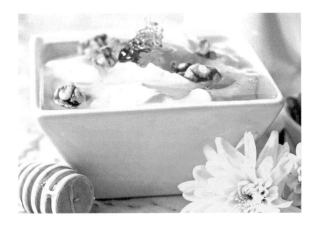

Over the Greek yoghurt, drizzle some honey.

To modify for sweetness, start with a few teaspoons and work your way up.

Add your preferred fresh fruit, sliced peaches, banana slices or berries.

For a little more crunch and flavour, sprinkle in chopped nuts, such as walnuts or almonds.

Optional garnish:
Add a few mint leaves as a garnish if you'd like to add some freshness.

Mix the ingredients together gently, being careful to spread the honey evenly.

Serve your honey-flavoured Greek yoghurt for a filling and tasty breakfast, snack or dessert.

You may easily alter the recipe to suit your tastes by substituting dried fruits, granola or chia seeds for some of the toppings.

Rice Cake with Avocado

Ingredients:

- One rice cake *(choose your preferred kind)*
- 1 ripe avocado
- *To taste*, Salt and pepper.

- Red pepper flakes, sesame seeds, lime juice or your preferred herbs - *optional garnishes.*

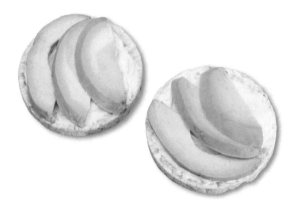

Instruction:

Halve the ripe avocado and scoop out the pit. Put the avocado flesh into a bowl using a spoon.

Mash the avocado with a fork until the consistency you want is achieved. It may be left quite lumpy or smoothed out.

Put some seasoning on the avocado.

To taste, add more salt and pepper. *For added taste*, you may also squeeze in some lime juice.

Evenly distribute the mashed avocado over the rice cake.

Over the mashed avocado, sprinkle your preferred toppings. You might use fresh herbs for extra freshness, sesame seeds for texture or red pepper flakes for a hint of fire.

It's now time to eat your avocado-topped rice cake.
It's a light supper or a fast, healthful snack

You may easily alter the recipe to suit your tastes by topping it with poached eggs, radishes or cherry tomatoes.

MEAL PLANNER FOR DIFFERENT DIETARY NEEDS.

DIET PLANNER
What I'll be Eating]

	BREAKFAST	LUNCH	DINNER	SNACKS
MON				
TUE				
WED				
THUR				
FRI				
SAT				
SUN				

DIET PLANNER
What I'll be Eating]

	BREAKFAST	LUNCH	DINNER	SNACKS
MON				
TUE				
WED				
THUR				
FRI				
SAT				
SUN				

DIET PLANNER
What I'll be Eating]

	BREAKFAST	LUNCH	DINNER	SNACKS
MON				
TUE				
WED				
THUR				
FRI				
SAT				
SUN				

Have A Safe And Speedy

RECOVERY ℰ

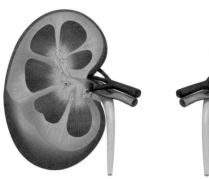
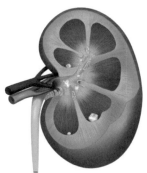